Loose weight without dieting working out

By

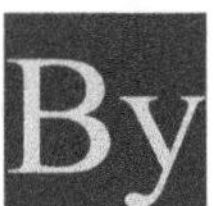

Scott scholz

Introduction

Starting on a weight loss journey might sound daunting if you're someone who doesn't love to hit the gym. While physical activity has many positive benefits for your health, it's just one piece of the puzzle regarding losing weight.

Luckily, if you cannot make it to the gym, there are many other ways to lose weight within a realistic timeline that don't involve lifting dumbbells or jogging on the treadmill. No matter what reason you have for starting a weight loss journey, implementing a few changes in your daily routine can help you on the path to better health, primarily if you've found it challenging to lose weight in the past.

Can You Lose Weight Without Exercising?

The simple answer is yes—there are many weight loss strategies that can be effective, and exercising is only one of them. Exercising in some forms, like strength training, can be a helpful tool to help you speed up your metabolic rate and burn some extra calories, but there are other simple practices you can implement into your lifestyle that can also give you an extra boost. Making changes to your diet, getting adequate sleep, and better understanding how stress is impacting your body can all be helpful in supporting weight loss for some people.

If you are looking for the fastest way to lose weight without exercise, it's important to note that while weight loss drugs like Ozempic and Wegovy have recently risen in popularity for their often quick results, there are still certain safety concerns being revealed by researchers as it pertains to their use. An October 2023 study found that drugs like Ozempic may lead to serious digestive problems, and other research has found that those who lose weight using GLP-1 drugs often regain it after stopping the medication.

Luckily, there are various daily lifestyle changes you can

implement that can help support sustainable, long-term weight loss. So, whether you're unable to exercise or you simply would prefer not to, here are 20 of the best ways to lose weight without exercise.

1) <u>**Start Your Meals With Protein**</u>

Breaking your overnight fast with a source of <u>high-quality protein</u> has been shown to help with satiety and blood sugar management. It may even help with diet quality in individuals with obesity.

Pairing <u>carbohydrates with protein</u> can also help to curb glucose spikes when eating, which is especially important after a fast since the protein helps slow the release of glucose from the carbohydrates into your bloodstream.

Keeping your glucose regulated may be helpful for weight management since insulin resistance may lead to weight gain over time. Focus on including high-quality protein sources in your diet, such as poultry, fatty fish, plain Greek yogurt, grass-fed meats, tofu, and tempeh for optimal blood sugar response.

Apart from preventing glucose spikes after a fast, there are many studies out there to demonstrate the connection between high-protein diets and weight loss. Protein is essential for muscle-building, promotes satietythroughout the day, and may help reduce excessive snacking.

2) <u>Watch Your Portion Sizes</u>

If you've struggled with your weight while eating a nutritious, whole foods-based diet, your <u>portion sizes</u>might be why you haven't seen the number on the scale decrease. While this may seem obvious, nutritional information on products can sometimes be misleading or difficult to interpret. Studies have shown that exposure <u>to </u>

<u>large portions</u> can lead to weight gain, so focusing on portion control and how much food is on your plate is essential.

Individuals who <u>struggle with obesity can benefit</u> from learning how to independently judge portion sizes when seeking to lose weight. Using smaller plates is one simple way to make portion control a little easier.

3) <u>Stay Hydrated</u>

Drinking enough water to support adequate hydration has been associated with weight loss through a few mechanisms. Some studies show that drinking water can help reduce calorie intake, making weight management that much easier.

Remember that staying hydrated isn't only beneficial for weight loss. It also can help reduce your risk of developing conditions like diabetes, cancer,

Alzheimer's, and <u>many other chronic diseases</u>. For tips to help you get adequate fluids throughout the day, check out our article on the importance of proper hydration.

4) <u>Reduce Added Sugar</u>

It might be one of the most common things you've heard if you have tried dieting for weight loss, and for a good reason. Excess sugar intake is one of the <u>leading causes of obesity</u> in the United States. Although eating junk food and sweets can be enjoyable, these foods are often high in <u>calories, added sugar, and trans fat</u>, meaning that cutting them out of your diet can significantly impact weight loss and overall health.

Fortunately, limiting extra sugars and processed foods with saturated fats has many other benefits besides weight loss. These dietary changes may support healthier skin and better triglyceride and cholesterol levels as well as help prevent other chronic conditions.

5) <u>Consider Testing Your Caffeine Tolerance</u>

Studies on the metabolic impacts of caffeine or coffee are conflicting. While some studies suggest that regular caffeine intake may be harmless or even helpful for some people, other studies show that it may cause elevations in cortisol and perhaps contribute to some other hormonal imbalances for certain people.

For those with diabetes, caffeine may make glucose control more difficult. However, it may slightly lower the risk for diabetes in those who aren't diabetic. Caffeine has a dose-dependent effect, which means that how it affects you may depend on the dose. Consider testing out different amounts or even taking a more extended break to assess how your body might respond to these different elements.

6) <u>Create a Symptom and Food Log</u>

Sometimes difficulty losing weight can be tied to underlying health imbalances and concerns. Tuning into how you *feel* is every bit as important, if not more important, than a number on a scale. Being able to identify symptoms of concern may help increase your awareness of how daily habits might be impacting how you're feeling.

Symptoms such as fatigue, anxiety, digestive upset, and poor sleep can sometimes offer added clues to metabolic imbalances. Tracking your personal symptom patterns over time, especially as you try new and different dietary approaches, can be an incredibly powerful tool to support you on your wellness journey.

Focusing on mindful eating and even using one of the various weight loss apps on the market can also help you create a schedule around eating and spot patterns more easily. Consider working one-on-one with a qualified nutritionist if you'd like more personalized support in this area.

7) <u>Avoid Sugary Drinks Like Soda or Juice</u>

We've already talked about the importance of reducing added sugar, but this one bears repeating. *"Don't drink your calories"* is a classic expression repeated in the weight loss space, and unfortunately, this includes soda, juice, alcohol, and most sugary drinks.

If you're cutting out some extra calories to help with your weight loss, these drinks do not provide much (if any) <u>nutritional value</u> and can be high in calories, which is why they are commonly referred to as "empty calories." By replacing these drinks with water, you'll not only be able to reap the health <u>benefits of being adequately hydrated</u>, but you'll also cut out some extra sugar and decrease the amount of empty calories you may be used to consuming.

8) <u>Get Plenty of Sleep</u>

Sleep is vital for many <u>aspects of your health</u>, including blood pressure, immune health, cognitive function, diabetes risk, cardiovascular disease, and more. That's why it's no surprise that insufficient sleep can have a <u>negative impact</u> on individuals with obesity.

Chronic sleep deprivation can also make other weight-loss tactics less effective over time, which is why getting plenty of rest is one of the crucial foundations of healthy weight loss. Prioritizing sleep by heading to bed 30 minutes to an hour earlier each night is a great way to get started.

9) <u>Eat More Non-Starchy Vegetables</u>

Including lots of non-starchy vegetables in your diet is rarely bad (as long as you tolerate them), and it's proven to be particularly beneficial when it comes to weight loss. Studies have shown that <u>increasing vegetable consumption led to measurable weight loss</u> in healthy individuals and also helped lower the risk of weight gain.

Vegetables are full of nutritious vitamins, minerals, and fiber and are generally low in calories, making them an excellent healthy snack for people looking to lose weight. Try pairing carrot or bell pepper slices with protein like hummus for a quick and satiating snack.

10) Limit Alcohol Consumption

Alcohol can lead
to inflammation in the body and
is another common source of
empty calories. It has also
been linked to overeating, so
it's only natural that limiting
your intake of beer, wine, and
spirits can be beneficial for
weight loss.

Studies have shown that
reducing alcohol consumption
was linked to weight loss in
overweight individuals. At the

same time, excessive alcohol intake may also be a <u>risk factor for obesity</u>, so it's best to limit your drinks if you're on a weight loss journey.

11) <u>Use Healthier Cooking Ingredients</u>

Swapping out unhealthier fat options for healthier cooking alternatives like olive oil, avocado oil, or coconut oil can be helpful for weight loss and have a range of other positive health effects. While all cooking oils are high in calories and fat, olive oil and coconut oil may have healthier effects on cholesterol levels and have no significant associations with increased mortality, unlike options like margarine.

One study among women with breast cancer found that a diet enriched with olive oil brought about more weight loss than a standard low-fat diet, showing the positive association of this type of oil on health.

12) Eat Without Distractions

If you're someone who is always watching TV with dinner or looking at your phone while you eat lunch, you may want to try putting your devices down during meals. Research shows that distracted eating may lead to overeating, which is linked to weight gain.

That's why mindful eating, or eating slowly can be beneficial when it comes to weight loss. Studies suggest that eating your food slowly can lead to increased satiety, or make you feel full faster. Aim to chew your food thoroughly and pace yourself while eating to support your weight loss journey.

13) Limit Emotional Stress

Many of the items in our list so far have to do with limiting stress of many kinds. Stress can come in the form of nutrient imbalances, poor sleep, and even alcohol consumption. But stress also comes in the form of psychosocial or what some people consider an "emotional" form.

When you experience high-stress levels or chronic stress of any kind, you may notice that you feel physically sick. Chronic stress is a risk factor for obesity and type 2 diabetes, among many other health concerns - which is why practicing relaxation techniques can be beneficial.

Stress can have a direct impact on your glucose levels and can even lead to insulin resistance over time. Taking steps to reduce stress can benefit more than just weight management. It can also help your mental health, support better sleep, and reduce your risk for chronic health conditions.

14) Cook More—Carry Out & Dine Out Less

Ordering take-out may be more convenient, especially if you're busy during the week or don't enjoy cooking. Unfortunately, many restaurants use excess butter, oil, and fat, adding many extra calories to your meal. There's also a chance you'll eat larger portions than usual, often exceeding recommended serving sizes.

Because of this, studies have found a link between eating home-cooked meals frequently and better overall health, including lower cholesterol, better metabolic health, and a lower risk of obesity. Eating at home more frequently can help you better control your calorie and macronutrient intake, may help with weight control, and even save money.

15) Weigh Yourself Regularly

This may not seem like a weight loss tip, per se. But it is! When you set realistic goals, you are more likely to stick to your path and avoid feelings of overwhelm that might lead to giving up before you hit your goal. Keep in mind that it's normal for your weight to fluctuate by a few pounds depending on factors like time of day, hydration level, and exercise.

If you're using a scale to track your progress, try to weigh yourself at an interval that doesn't feel too triggering and focus on how you're feeling first and foremost. Keeping track of your weight changes may be helpful but over-focusing on weighing yourself or weighing yourself too often may just add more stress to your plate.

16) Stand, Stretch, & Walk During the Day

Taking time to stand up often throughout the day, get some extra steps in, or even stretch have also been linked to increased weight loss. Standing burns <u>more calories than sitting</u>; while it may sound insignificant, these calories can add up over time.

Walking and <u>other activities</u> you may do throughout the day have been shown to be <u>positive for overall health</u> and can play a big role in weight management over time by keeping you moving and getting your heart rate up.

17) <u>Prioritize Your Fiber Intake</u>

There are numerous health benefits of fiber, including supporting gut health, blood sugar regulation, and cardiovascular health. But not only that, including an appropriate amount of fiber in your diet can even support healthy weight loss.

Including fiber-rich foods in your meals can keep you satiated and feeling full for longer, and it can help reduce inflammation in the body, which is linked to weight gain. The Dietary Guidelines for Americans recommendconsuming 22 to 34 grams of fiber per day depending on factors like age and sex. Good sources of fiber include whole grains, non-starchy veggies, beans, legumes, nuts, and seeds.

Bonus tip: Eat your fiber first alongside your protein and before your carbs to help slow your body's digestion of any carbs or sugars in your meal to help keep your blood sugar balanced.

18) Focus on Whole Foods and Reduce Ultra-Processed Foods

Eating a balanced, whole foods-based diet has many potential health benefits, one of which is weight loss. Whole foods are nutrient-rich and promote satiety. When you focus on whole foods, you may naturally eat fewer simple carbohydrates, ultra-processed foods, and added sugars that can lead to weight gain and overeating. Here are a few examples of whole food sources from each macronutrient group to try adding to your diet.

Whole Carbohydrates

Focus on red or sweet potatoes, low-glycemic fruits, vegetables, whole grains like quinoa and steel cut oats, beans, and legumes.

Whole Proteins

These can come from chicken, fish, eggs, plain Greek yogurt, grass-fed meats, and tofu.

Whole Fats

Try to include a variety of foods such as avocados, nuts, seeds, fatty fish, and olives. Most animal proteins also contain whole sources of fat.

19) Create a Plan for Emotional Eating

Emotional eating is often associated with weight gain. If you find yourself using food to cope with emotions or want to cut down on snacking throughout the day, creating a meal plan and schedule that you can stick to is a great way to hold yourself accountable.

You may also try keeping a food journal and keeping track of the emotions you feel when you experience cravings to help you explore some deeper motivators driving your meal choices.

20) <u>Utilize a Standing Desk</u>

Being sedentary has several negative health effects, and as we already know, standing more often throughout the day can be <u>beneficial for weight loss</u>. If you have the option, trying out a standing or height-adjustable desk is just one way to spend less time sitting if you have a sedentary job.

One study found that using a standing desk didn't significantly impact work performance, meaning that this alternative to sitting might be helpful to try. Standing desks may also support lower blood pressure and less lower back pain. However, more research is still needed to determine the correlation.

Engage with Your Blood Glucose Levels with Nutrisense

Your blood sugar levels can significantly impact how your body feels and functions. That's why stable blood glucose levels can be an important factor in supporting overall wellbeing.

With Nutrisense, you'll be able to track your blood glucose levels over time using a CGM, so you can make lifestyle choices that support healthy living.

When you join the Nutrisense CGM program, our team of credentialed dietitians and nutritionists are available for additional support and guidance to help you reach your goals.

Ready to take the first step? Start with our quiz to see how Nutrisense can support your health.

www.ingramcontent.com/pod-product-compliance
Lightning Source LLC
Chambersburg PA
CBHW080944260726
48661CB00010B/4078